Ethical Practices in Yoga

How Yama and Niyama help make a better you

The School of Yoga 4

Anand Gupta

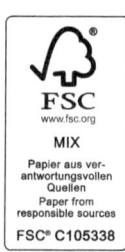

Bibliografische Information der Deutschen Nationalbibliothek:

Die Deutsche Nationalbibliothek verzeichnet diese Publikation in der Deutschen Nationalbibliografie; detaillierte bibliografische Daten sind im Internet über http://dnb.dnb.de abrufbar.

© 2020, Anand Gupta, 2nd Edition

Herstellung und Verlag: BoD –
Books on Demand, Norderstedt

ISBN: 978-3-7526-2283-6

Introduction

By using this book, you accept this disclaimer in full.

No advice

The book contains information. The information is not advice and should not be treated as such.

No representations or warranties

To the maximum extent permitted by applicable law and subject to section below, we exclude all representations, warranties, undertakings and guarantees relating to the book.

Without prejudice to the generality of the foregoing paragraph, we do not represent, warrant, undertake or guarantee:

- that the information in the book is correct, accurate, complete or non-misleading.

- that the use of the guidance in the book will lead to any particular outcome or result.

Limitations and exclusions of liability

The limitations and exclusions of liability set out in this section and elsewhere in this disclaimer: are subject to section 6 below; and govern all liabilities arising under the disclaimer or in relation to the book, including liabilities arising in contract, in tort (including negligence) and for breach of statutory duty.

We will not be liable to you in respect of any losses arising out of any event or events beyond our reasonable control.

We will not be liable to you in respect of any business losses, including without limitation loss of or damage to profits, income, revenue, use, production, anticipated savings, business, contracts, commercial opportunities or goodwill.

We will not be liable to you in respect of any loss or corruption of any data, database or software.

We will not be liable to you in respect of any special, indirect or consequential loss or damage.

Exceptions

Nothing in this disclaimer shall: limit or exclude our liability for death or personal injury resulting from negligence; limit or exclude our liability for fraud or fraudulent misrepresentation; limit any of our liabilities in any way that is not permitted under applicable law; or exclude any of our liabilities that may not be excluded under applicable law.

Severability

If a section of this disclaimer is determined by any court or other competent authority to be unlawful and/or unenforceable, the other sections of this disclaimer continue in effect.

If any unlawful and/or unenforceable section would be lawful or enforceable if part of it were deleted, that part will be deemed to be deleted, and the rest of the section will continue in effect.

Law and jurisdiction

This disclaimer will be governed by and construed in accordance with Swiss law, and any disputes relating to this disclaimer will be subject to the exclusive jurisdiction of the courts of Switzerland.

Inhaltsverzeichnis

Inhaltsverzeichnis	9
Introduction	**12**
Chapter 1: What is Ashtanga Yoga?	**14**
Yama and Niyama	*17*
Chapter 2: The Rules of Yama	**21**
Ahimsa or Non-violence	*22*
Satya or Truthfulness	*25*
Asteya or Non-stealing	*28*
Brahmacharya or Self-control	*30*
Aparigraha or Lacking the wish to hoard	*32*
Chapter 3: The Rules of Niyama	**34**
Shaucha or Purification	*35*
Santosha or Contentment	*36*
Tapas or Asceticism	*37*
Svadhyaya or Self-study	*38*
Ishvara pranidhana or Surrendering to one's destiny	*39*
Chapter 4: Importance of Yama and Niyama	**40**

Conclusion 48

Introduction

You've probably heard of Yoga and its benefits in general, and it is all through the practices of the different asanas alone. But as any passionate yoga instructor will tell you, the yoga is not whole without the spiritual and ethical disciplines to guide you, to discriminate the self from objects, to achieve spiritual enlightenment, to push you to achieve the union of mind and body which is the ultimate goal of Yoga. And the very first step in this direction is in understanding *what not to do*. This is defined under the Yamas, which is the very first step in the Ashtanga yoga (also called Eight-limbed Yoga or Raja yoga), followed by the rules that define *what is to be done* which are listed under the Niyamas. The asanas make up the third aspect of the Ashtanga Yoga.

Before we discuss the Yamas and Niyamas in Yoga, we need to properly understand what is Raja Yoga or Ashtanga Yoga and how it incorporates these rules.

Chapter 1: What is Ashtanga Yoga?

Patanjali was the first person to codify the age old concept and practices of Yoga in around 400 C.E. The *Pātañjalayogaśāstra,* or the Yoga Sutras of Patanjali presents the best (raja) of the Yogic practices, taking notes from older traditions as well as Patanjali's own commentary.

From Patanjali's work, the concept of Ashtanga system of Yoga is derived. This word if coined from the words Ashta ('eight') and anga ('limbs'), this literally meaning 'eight-limbs'. The Ashtanga or Eight-limbed Yoga is designed to make you reach enlightenment, through breathing practice and meditation on the move. The guiding practices and observances listed within this form of Yoga are meant to help the Yogi achieve the state of consciousness that is free from all thoughts and eventually helping the Yogi to attentively discern between what is essential and what is non-essential, what is self and what is not-self, as defined by the complete discriminative knowledge. Thus, it is a path to spiritual awakening of self through patience, perseverance, discipline and commitment.

The eight limbs of this form of Yoga mentioned in the Yogasutra of Patanjali are:

- *Yama* (also known as the list of universal vows) is a list of don't-dos or restraints.

- *Niyama* is a set of dos that enables a yogi to conserve the energy he or she gets from observing the restraints.

- *Asana* are the postures that help a yogi to meditate, balance and harmonize the body and mind.

- *Pranayama* explains the breath regulation. But it is not just about controlling the breath but also your energy.

- *Pratyahara* is the withdrawal of senses from external world. It is an art of controlling your senses, life force and actions in order to withdraw or detach the mind from the external surroundings.

- *Dharana* is concentration. It is the art of applying concentration in any given task and doing it with happiness or contentment, without feeling the burden and pain of it.

- *Dhyana* is abstract meditation. It involves achieving a state of mind where the yogi's body and mind are detached from the objects and events in their environment, so that he or she is able to ignore any distraction in the surroundings effortlessly and attain mental bliss.

- *Samadhi* is oneness: the state of perfected concentration, wherein the Yogi finds his true self and becomes one with it.

Though it is one of the hardest forms of Yoga, the Ashtanga is beneficial not only for physical health but also for attaining mental clarity and awareness, as well as harmony with self and the world. Instead of focusing plainly on the physical practices of Yoga, dare to go beyond and couple it with its spiritual essence to reap further benefits for yourself.

Yama and Niyama

Yama in Yoga

The Rig Veda and many earlier texts mention and discuss the word Yamas. Etymologically, within the context of the Rig Veda the word Yamas means a rein or a curb, or the act of restraining as done by a charioteer. In the later scriptures, the usage of the word evolved to mean a moral restraint or self discipline or forbearance. In Patanjali's Yoga

Sutras, the first limb or rung of Eight Limbed Yoga, or Ashtanga Yoga, is the Yamas. There are five Yamas that define a set of restraints and abstinences for a Yogi to follow in order to lead a virtuous life. These ethical principles must be practiced by the Yogi when he or she is in the external world and also while interacting with people. The purpose behind following these restrictions is in not only to help one in nurturing better relationship with their environment and people, but also in understanding how our relationship with the world and people eventually affects us and our ability to achieve self realization. The focus of these principles is to help the Yogi achieve personal fulfilment all the while enabling him or her to benefit the society as well. The yamas are used to harness the energy the yogi can otherwise waste in other actions. The energy saved by these restrictions can be directed by the Yogi for any better purpose that serves as a means to achieve spiritual awakening.

Niyama in Yoga

Niyama is the secondary rung or limb of the Ashtanga and is complimentary to the Yama. Within the context of Yoga, the niyama, in contrast to Yama, is a set of "dos" that a Yogi can observe for a virtuous and healthy lifestyle. The niyama lists rules that help a Yogi to conserve the energy that is gathered through the practice of restraints or yama. These rules are self disciplinatory and instil virtues habits in a yogi.

Together, Yama and Niyama make up the rules and goals for a Yogi to practice in order to set an ideal lifestyle. The practicing of Yamas help us to conserve our energy through a peaceful life whereas the practicing of Niyamas help us foster dedication through effectively utilizing this conserved energy. The ultimate goal is to achieve a healthier lifestyle. These practices are not easy to follow and can only be incorporated in your life slowly, through patience and perseverance. Call on these practices when you feel something that goes against their principle and enable yourself to strengthen and fortify your mind and your relationship with your environment.

Chapter 2: The Rules of Yama

The five Yamas listed in the Patanjali's Yogasutra are:

Ahimsa: Non-violence, not hurting or harming others

Satya: Truth, Being honest, not lying

Asteya: Not stealing, abstaining from thievery

Brahmacharya: Expressing the dharma, practicing self control through remembrance of the Higher being

Aparigraha: Freedom from covetousness, Lacking greed or indulgence

The purpose of the practice of Yamas is detailed below:

Ahimsa or Non-violence

ahiṁsā pratiṣṭhāyāṁ tat samnidhau vaira tyāgaḥ - When non-violence is firmly established in a Yogi, every conflict with the environment is naturally abandoned.

The first Yama in Yoga is Ahimsa. The Sanskrit word 'ahimsa' generally means restraint from harming or showing impertinence to any living creature and in any way, whether it is physical, mental or emotional. However, within the context of Yoga, ahimsa is a concept beyond restraining from aggressive behaviour towards others. Yoga is focussed on helping on establish unity between mind, body and soul. Ahimsa for a Yogi is a means of restraining from harming oneself, through interactions with other people or things, and how this restraint eventually helps him or her benefit by being cautious beforehand. Ahimsa is about creating a cautious mentality instead of a judgemental or critical one and thus avoiding any acts of violence by display or anger or irritation. A yogi must not hurt anyone or anything, either by his or her thoughts, words and actions. The philosophy of ahimsa preaches that a Yogi's firmness in non-violence will naturally enable other living beings or creatures in his or her environment to withdraw their hostility towards him or her, thus creating peace around themselves.

Any hostility or impatience within one self will naturally prevents him or her from attaining peace with everything. For example, as a yogi you must meditate with a peaceful mind and within a space that allows you to adhere to this peace. You cannot meditate properly should you carry any thoughts (excitement or fears) within your mind or your place of meditation creates distractions for you. Firmly seating the ahimsa within yourself will enable you to practise your yoga in any setting, thus freeing yourself from the notions of threats, by the lack of its acknowledgement, and the fears that come with it. Your personal vibe of peacefulness will deter any possible threat away from you. Only by letting go of the negative feelings of hostility and violence can you beget peace for yourself. This in turn will allow you to create a circle of positivity and harmlessness in your surroundings. Thus, ahimsa not only benefits you but every living thing that comes in contact with you.

Ahimsa is fostered with compassion towards others, may it be people or living creatures. Training yourself to accept everything as it is the first step to being compassionate. Refrain from negatively reacting to events and keep an open mind and a loving heart. Replace your negative thoughts and feelings with positive ones: tell yourself how things can be good this way too, remind yourself of how kindness can change things, train yourself to accept the events as they occur. Nurture peace within yourself and watch it expand outwards, through you and into your environment.

Satya or Truthfulness

satya pratiṣṭhāyāṁ kriyā phalā 'śrayatvaṁ - When the state of being truthful is firmly established in a Yogi, every (truthful) action is found to have a supporting result.

The second Yama in Yoga is Satya. Satya means Truth and within the understanding of Yoga, it is a notion of discussing the truth and holding on to truth through your actions. But satya must not be such that it induces violence within the environment. Instead, a Yogi must be able to visibly perceive what the truth is, so that every action that he or she undertakes will eventually result in a reaction that is equally fruitful. Satya is the state of being truthfully aware, of having a clear vision on how to intelligently handle the situations so that every action and reaction is linked with each other in their outcome. Your good intentions should yield you good results. As a yogi, you must be aware of how your words and deeds affect everything or everyone else in your surroundings.

As a person who establishes satya, you will create a level of respect and honour for yourself in the eyes of others. As a yogi with well established satya, you will see through your every action with utmost honesty and naturally will it into a result of your choice. The essence of satya is in having your heart and lips adhere to the same truth.

As a yogi, teach yourself to refrain from lying, as the very act disconnects you from your higher self. Your lies will instil both distrust and fear of others, and before long you will realize that you cannot trust yourself too. By adhering to satya you can set yourself free by the simple act of self realization. Being honest with yourself is as important as keeping honesty with others.

Although the major idea of Satya is to encourage a Yogi to live a truthful life and speak truthfully at all the times, it is also deemed necessary to have your satya should project your ahimsa. If your action is likely to cause negativity then it is appropriate to abandon it rather than cause a violent stir. This does not mean that you can lie, but it is advisable to withhold your tongue from making any statements to maintain peace and refrain from harming others. Sense the truth as it is, rather than thinking about it. Satya is not practiced by analyzing or assuming the truth or by reasoning for it.

Asteya or Non-stealing

asteya pratiṣṭhāyāṁ sarva ratna u'pasthānaṁ - When the non-stealing has been firmly established in a Yogi, every treasure is made available near to him.

The third Yama in Yoga is Asteya. Asteya teaches a yogi to not steal from others or take advantage of them for your own benefit, given their trust and confidence in you. A yogi must not take anything that is not freely offered to him or her, neither should the yogi encourage others in doing so. Asteya is not only practiced with respect to articles, but with words too. It is not deemed appropriate to present other's words or ideas as your own. Your good character is manifested by making proper acknowledgements where it is required. You need to be honest when you deal with others, irrespective of what you exchange with them and how you exchange it.

Asteya encourages a yogi to refrain from exploiting other people, creatures or environment for personal benefit. In other words, it prevents them from oppressing others or being unjust towards them. You need to free yourself from desire of other things in order to save yourself from hoarding. You need to be content with what you already have, what you earn for yourself and what you get from others, instead of pondering over what you want but do not have as this will very likely lead you to think about stealing it from others who do.

Through Asteya a Yogi can overcome his or her greed. Asteya can be practiced by being generous to others and giving away instead of hoarding. Learn to share your possessions with others and in return you will doubly benefit.

Brahmacharya or Self-control

brahmacarya pratiṣṭhāyāṁ vīrya lābhaḥ - When every action is firmly performed with awareness of an absolute truth by a Yogi, it leads to vital strength.

The fourth Yama in Yoga is Brahmacharya. Brahmacharya is an act that promotes abstinence from energetic actions or emotions; it helps a Yogi to direct the movement of their energy in a single direction rather than several directions. A person normally dissipates his or her energy in emotions such as anger, lust etc. The practice of abstinence helps a yogi conserve his or her energy which is generally wasted through thoughts, words or actions, thus helping them perform their actions effortlessly with a singular focus. The foremost idea of abstinence is to control one's impulses that are of physical nature and instead act responsibly with others and towards our environment. Only be controlling these impulses can we understand our addictions and how we can curb them, thus enabling ourselves to be more vigorous. Each addiction that we overcome builds up our courage to overcome others and adds a reserve of strength to our beings. Only through abstinence can we free ourselves from the mental and physical restrictions that are bound to us through our senses and achieve the inner balance as well as the awareness of a higher reality.

Brahmacharya primarily stresses on celibacy to conserve the energy we dissipate in physical or mental form of sexual activity. This energy can be utilized for enlightening oneself with awareness of self and others as living beings, for creating an environment of harmony and fidelity. The philosophy of Brahmacharya is to achieve sobriety with respect to the surroundings through remembrance of the divine.

Aparigraha or Lacking the wish to hoard

aparigrahasthairye janma kathantā sambodhaḥ - When the lack of covetousness (or hoarding) is firmly established in a Yogi, the need for knowledge of the mysteries (why and how) of life and its goal arises

The last yama in Yoga is known as Aparigraha. Aparigraha encompasses the concepts of lacking avarice or covetousness and being content with life. A Yogi must learn to let go of what is not needed by him and be content with what he or she possess, as little as it may be for objects in this world cannot be kept in possession for long and are subject to destruction. Avarice hampers our ability to connect with our true self and acknowledge the purpose of our being and our existence. The fear of loss of worldly possessions restricts us from gaining independence. Aparigraha teaches a Yogi to detach themselves from the things in their life so that their loss does not make them miserable or wretched. If you focus your energy on many things then you cannot achieve one real purpose.

Chapter 3: The Rules of Niyama

The five Niyamas given by Patanjali in the Yogasutras are:

Shaucha: Purity of mind and body, Cleanliness, Hygiene

Santosha: Contentment, Mental comfort, Satisfaction, Happiness

Tapas: Self discipline, asceticism

Svadhyaya: Studying one's self, Reflecting on sacred words

Ishvara pranidhana: Surrendering to one's destiny

The Niyamas benefit the Yogi as given below:

Shaucha or Purification

śaucāt svā 'ṅga jugupsā parair asaṁsargaḥ - Purity of one's own body results in dissociation with other things.

sattva śuddhi saumanasyai 'kāgrye 'ndriya jayā 'tma darśana yogyatvāni ca – And, the habit of cleanliness, as well as the mastery over the senses, leads to self realization

The first Niyama in Yoga is the Shaucha. The principle indicates that the presence of any form of impurity withIn our body or in our surroundings will ultimately create adverse effects in our mind and its state. Thus this impurity will prevent us from properly attaining wisdom through self realization. Our spiritual awakening is only made possible with our habit of maintaining hygiene with ourselves and our surroundings, as well as attaining mastery over our senses, otherwise they can hinder us from keeping focus and mental clarity. The goal of yoga is to enable a yogi to live a healthy life and maintaining cleanliness of body and purity of mind for ones' self is the first step in that direction. Thus the first niyama focuses on purity and the habit of maintaining it, so that the yogi can develop mental harmony with self and environment.

Santosha or Contentment

saṁtoṣād anuttamaḥ sukha lābhaḥ - Contentment gives rise to unparalleled joy

The second niyama in yoga is Santosha. Santosha encourages the yogi to be satisfied with his or her possessions, materialistic or not, instead of craving for things that do not belong to them, as self satisfaction and contentment can only lead to unbound happiness and mental comfort. By coveting the possessions of others, we allow ourselves to project our energy in other directions and as such loose our focus and mental clarity. Being content with all that we have, all that we are and all that life gives us is the shortest way to achieve true joy. The greed for worldly objects can only provide us with a temporary happiness, but contentment is an everlasting feeling as it is rooted in positivity. Through santosha a yogi expresses his or her gratitude and is free to acknowledge the joys and blessings in their life. Santosha frees us from feeling negatively and suffering as a result of these emotions. With santosha, a yogi is liberated from unnecessarily wanting things.

Tapas or Asceticism

kāye 'ndriya siddhir aśuddhi kṣayāt tapasaḥ - Self discipline destroys mental impurities and thus, the body and inner senses attain perfection

The third niyama in yoga is Tapas or self discipline. Through tapas, the yogi seek to discipline themselves and enhance their will power. Through tapas, a yogi wills himself to achieve any task and gain a positive outcome for it through determination to see it through and dedication to get it done. Tapas is the redirection of one's energy into positive work by fighting against one's urges or desires.

Svadhyaya or Self-study

svādhyāyād iṣṭa devatā samprayogaḥ - Self-study and reflection unites one with the desired divinity

Svadhyaya is the power to see through ourselves, understand and reflect on life in order to realize what we seek and bring ourselves closer to that goal. Svadhyaya involves learning lessons from not only our own life and its mistakes, but from our ideals, in order to clearly see ourselves and our connection with the divine.

Ishvara pranidhana or Surrendering to one's destiny

samādhi siddhir īśvara praṇidhānāt – Self realization is attained by accepting one's fate

Ishvara pranidhana is the fifth and last niyama of Yoga. It is the devotion to a higher being and the acceptance of one's fate, of how one's dedicated practice brings them closer to their what they want. The practice of yoga is attuned with a person's need to connect with the higher being and attain self realization through the ensuing spiritual awakening. The first step in this path is to let go of the egocentric self, to accept the higher being and devote our time and energy to it.

Chapter 4: Importance of Yama and Niyama

The Yamas and the Niyamas are a set of rules that define the "dos" and "don't dos" in order to achieve an ideal Yogic life. But these age old rules not only benefit a person within the sphere of Yoga but also beyond that and into our modern lives. The Yamas teach us how cultivating the opposite of what the self urges us to do will yield us more benefits, whereas the Niyamas lists the observances for better self training.

Within the context of Yoga, each rule enables the Yogi to unfold some ability during meditation. Beginning with the first Yama – ahimsa – a yogi's own personal vibe of peace will enable others in his or her surrounding to bring out the peace within themselves. It also enables the yogi to safely detach themselves from his or her environment and carry on with their practice in a blissful state of mind. Being non-violent towards yourself is where to start your practice: yoga is not about getting your postures right, but about attaining that inner peace and unity of body and mind. Ahimsa allows you to bring peace to your yoga practice. Instead of racing through the postures just to ensure your flexibility to yourself or occupying your thoughts in wondering if your postures are graceful or perfect, use ahimsa to clear your mind and bring it peace as you mediate and perform your asanas. Keep to your personal space at a distance that allows you to freely practice your asanas without interfering with others.

You can maintain satya on your yoga mat by adhering to your purpose to achieve the mental stability. Acknowledge your own limitations, how much you can push yourself. Stay truthful about your progress or lack of it with yourself and others: you are not expected to achieve the hardest of the asanas in the very first week of your practice, nor are you expected to be an expert yogi if you've had years of practice. Stop yourself from being judgemental or critical of yourselves or others.

Practice Asteya through your punctuality; organize your time so that you are well in advance for the practice and have enough time for some warm ups. Throughout the session utilize your time effectively in achieving or trying to achieve the postures, and do not let your mind ponder over what else you need to do, where you need to be next. Be accepting of who you are and what you can do rather than try to mask it just because you feel out of shape or practice or are not in the mood. Do not interfere with others' space or mental peace, including the instructor. Bring abstinence with you by maintaining your patience during the class and directing your energy to achieving the asanas rather than letting your mind and eyes wander here and there. Keenly follow the instructions as given by the instructor to ensure you are directing your energy properly. Detach yourself from your surroundings to ensure you are following the principle of Aparigraha. Focus on your breathing and postures instead.

Maintain your hygiene and cleanliness. Wear proper and clean clothes when you go to the studio; choose the ones you are comfortable with during the yoga practice. It is better to bring your own yoga practice mat to the session and choose a spot that is clean and pleasant in ambience. Be content with your own practice and what you achieved during the session; do not compare yourself with others and how their postures are more graceful and fluidic than yours. This will only cause you to cultivate negativity within yourself. Tune yourself out from your surroundings and only let yourself be guided by the instructions being relayed to you. The words of the instructor must be your beacon to attaining tapas, so let them evoke the passion to achieve the goal (or the posture) for you. Study yourself and your progress: what posture is difficult for you to do? Why is it difficult for you to achieve? How can you train yourself to achieve it? Pay attention to yourself and how you practice. Are you holding the posture right or is it just visibly right? How do you balance your weight and where do you hold the tension? Surrender your ego to the higher being or the Divine and let yourself unfold the true strength of your body through this devotion.

Besides your yoga mat, the principles of Yama and Niyama will equally benefit you in your day to day life. Ahimsa practiced through compassion with enable you to create a en environment of harmony and peace with the people in your life. If you make up your mind to refrain from showing any improper behaviour or acting aggressively in response to any event, you will have made a best example of yourself. You do not need to love everything, you only need to show and feel compassion towards it. Ahimsa teaches you to be mindful of your thoughts and actions before directing them towards any living creature. Satya is an important quality to have in order to maintain any relationship. It is not just about being truthful to yourself and others with your words and action, but about being aware of what your actions and words will yield back to you or portray to others. Let others build their trust with you by your honesty but make sure that you do not hurt others with your honesty too. This is followed up with Asteya, which asks you to refrain from thievery of any kind: objects or words. Do not let yourself feel inadequate as it is the root cause for any stealing, and also refrain from making others feel inadequate. Hoarding up objects unnecessarily is also another form of stealing where you constantly amass objects that could otherwise benefit others. Instead practice sharing or giving away your articles, properly acknowledging people with their rights as this will in turn add to your own karma and higher self.

Practice the behaviour that eventually leads you to the Divine path and devote your time to it for better self awareness. Direct your energies to setting up a positive environment and as such boosting your happiness and those of the others. Keep your surroundings tidy and maintain personal hygiene, as this will help you to create and maintain cleanliness not only where you live but also wherever you go. Keeping a check on cleanliness will allow you to positively connect with your environment and lend you the strength from it. A neat and tidy environment helps your mind to de-stress easily, unlike a cluttered environment that sets you up for feeling lazy. Find contentment with yourself and within yourself, so that you can find it with those around you and in your life. Fuel your passion for achieving your goals or showing creativity through sincere dedication to your work and a strong willpower.

Conclusion

In this book we have discussed the first two rungs or limbs of the Ashtanga Yoga or the Eight-limbed Yoga, and how they help one create balance and harmony not just within oneself but with their environment too. Yama presents a list of activities that must be avoided by a Yogi, or rather sets restrictions on the Yogi to ensure he or she develops a social restraint in order to make their relationship with their surroundings much better. The yamas listed in Patanjali's Yogasutra are: *non-violence, truthfulness, non-stealing, self-control* and *non-covetousness*. The Niyamas on the other hand are a set of observances that promote self discipline and improve will power. Yogasutra has the following niyamas: *purification, contentment, asceticism, self-study* and *surrender to destiny*. Together, these two moral imperatives help in bringing the Yogi closer to the goal of Yoga: unity of the body and mind. For a Yogi *now* is always the right time to start employing the rules of Yama and Niyama in their life. So don't wait till you are on the yoga mat or on your way to the next yoga session to work according to these rules. Begin now and improve your yoga practice as well as your social life by creating better interactions with the environment. Use the yamas to restrain yourself from any misdeed and save your energy; use the niyamas to positively utilize the energy for a better you.